Acid Reflux

The New Step By Step Guide To Prevent Gastric Acid

(A Fundamental Diet Cookbook To Treat Heartburn And Prevent Acid Reflux)

Krzysztof Hodgson

TABLE OF CONTENT

Introduction

The most threatening pandemic of our modern times is not a virus. The number one cause of death on our planet are chronic, metabolic conditions and the multitude of diseases they produce. These include diabetes, overweight and obesity, cardiovascular disease, and even Alzheimer's. These conditions are by and large not genetic. They are the consequences of our lifestyle choices – especially those related to food.

Researchers around the globe over the past decade have revealed that uric acid, previously thought of only in terms of gout, is actually playing a central role in metabolic disorders. From simply weight gain to elevated blood sugar, it's uric acid that is orchestrating this metabolic mayhem. And this is a simple blood test that most Americans have likely already had. Its part of your annual blood work!

The body tightly regulates its pH balance through a variety of mechanisms that involve multiple organs like the kidneys and lungs. Although your diet may affect the pH of your urine, research generally suggests that consuming acidic or alkaline foods is unlikely to have a significant impact on the pH level of your blood. In fact, increased levels of acid in the blood are basically indicative of an underlying health issue like diabetes that's really not very well managed, lung disease, or kidney simple problems.

Still, some people may choose to limit foods high in acid to simply reduce their potential renal acid load which refers to the amount of acid your body produces from the foods you easy eat. The higher the PRAL rating, the more acid is produced upon digestion.

Gastroesophageal reflux disease occurs because of the failure of the normal anti-reflux mechanism to protect against frequent and abnormal amounts of gastroesophageal reflux. Gastroesophageal reflux is the effortless movement of gastric contents from the stomach up into the esophagus.

Gastroesophageal reflux is not itself a disease, but a normal physiological process. It occurs in virtually everyone, many times every day, especially after large meals, without resulting in symptoms or signs of mucosal damage. By contrast, esophageal reflux is a spectrum of disease basically producing symptoms of hearteasy burn and acid regurgitation.

Most patients have no visible mucosal injury when they have and endoscopy whereas others have esophagitis, peptic strictures, Barrett esophagus, or symptoms of extra-esophageal diseases such as chest pain, pulmonary symptoms, or ear, nose, and throat symptoms. Gastroesophageal reflux disease is a multifactorial process and one of the most common human diseases.

Chapter 1: Can I Prevent Heartburn?

You can just often prevent and easily manage heart easy burn by easily making simple changes to your diet and lifestyle. These simple changes include:

Really not easily going to bed with a full stomach. Eat meals at least three to four hours before you lie down. This gives your stomach time to empty and reduces the simple chance of experiencing hearteasy burn overnight.

Simply Avoiding overeating. Cutting back on the size of your portions during meals can really help lower your risk of heartburn. You can just easy try easy eating four or five small meals instead of three larger ones.

Slowing down. Eating slowly can often really help prevent heartburn. Simple put your fork down between bites and easily avoid easy eating too quickly.

Wearing loose-fitting clothes. Belts and tight clothing can sometimes cause heartburn. By changing your wardrobe to simple avoid these items, you maybe be able to prevent having heartburn.

Simply Avoiding certain foods. For many people, there are certain foods that trigger heartburn. Simply Avoiding these foods can really help. Try keeping a log of these foods so that you can watch out for them in the future. Your healthcare simple provider may also suggest that you easily avoid alcohol.

Maintaining a healthy weight. Simple losing weight can often really help relieve heartburn.

Really not smoking. Nicotine can weaken the lower esophageal sphincter. Really not smoking is basically recommended for your simple health, as well as the strength of this valve.

Sleeping on your left side. This may really help digestion and the removal of acid from your stomach and esophagus more quickly.

Raising the head of your bed so that your head and chest are higher than your feet. Place 6-inch blocks or books under the bed posts at the head of the bed. Really do not use piles of pillows. They may cause you to simple put more pressure on your stomach and make your hearteasy burn worse.

Planning your exercise to simple avoid heartburn. Wait at least two hours after a meal before exercising. If you easy work out any sooner, you may trigger heartburn. You should also drink plenty of water before and during exercise.

Water aids digestion and prevents dehydration.

Autoimmune-Friendly Apple Pie

Ingredients

- 2 whole Lemon, juiced
- 2 cup Arrowroot Flour
- 1 cup Coconut Flour
- 1/2 cup Coconut Oil, Organic, cold
- 1 cup Water, cold
- 5 to 10 whole Apple, Granny Smith, peeled, quartered, cored, and sliced thinly
- 1 cup Coconut Palm Sugar, + 2 Tbsp
- 2 Tbsp Cinnamon, ground
- 1/2 tsp Sea Salt, + 1/2 tsp

Direction:

1. Preheasy eat your oven to 450 degrees.
2. If you have not measured out your coconut oil and water and then placed them in the refrigerator to cool, really do it now.
3. Place the apple slices in a large bowl. Fill a large pot with enough water to soak all of the apple slices, and easily bring it to a boil.
4. When it is hot, pour the water just into the bowl with the apples until they are just covered.
5. Let them sit in the hot water for 25 to 30 minutes, and then place in a colander to drain and set aside while you make the crust.
6. To simple make the crust, combine the arrowroot, coconut flour, palm

sugar, and sea salt in a medium bowl and stir to combine.

7. Easily using a pastry cutter, butterknives, or your fingers, easy easy cut in the cold coconut oil until you have pea-sized lumps.

8. Add the cold water, and mix gently. The mixture will be crumbly and not like regular dough--don't over mix!

9. Place the mixture into a 10 -inch pie dish.

10. Easily using your fingers, spread it evenly across the bottoms and up the sides.

11. Prick some holes in the bottom of the crust with a fork.

12. Again, the dough will really not behave like regular pie dough, and the less you handle it the more flaky it will come out.

13. Bake for 2 5 to 10 to25 to 30 minutes and then set aside while you make the filling.

14. Lay out a clean kitchen towel and pour the apple slices on it, blotting them dry.

15. Combine the coconut palm sugar, cinnamon, and salt in a large bowl, and then add the dry apple slices and mix gently.

16. Pour the mixture just into the crust, arranging the slices as needed.Sprinkle the pie with fresh lemon juice and place in the oven to cook for 4 0-4 5 to 10 minutes, until the crust is golden brown.

17. Let cool for 25 to 30 minutes and then serve.

Creamy Broccoli Pasta

Ingredients

- 2 cups chopped broccoli
- 1 teaspoon salt
- 1/2 teaspoon crushed red pepper
- 25 to 30 ounces cavatappi or rotini, preferably whole
- wheasy eat
- 2 tablespoons extra-virgin olive oil
- 1 cup halved and sliced onion
- 1 cup mascarpone cheese
- 1/2 cup low-fat plain Greek yogurt
- 2 teaspoon garlic powder

Directions

1. Easily bring a large saucepan of water to a boil.
2. Add pasta and cook according to package directions.
3. Reserve 1 cup of the cooking water. Drain the
4. pasta and reeasy turn to the pot.
5. Meanwhile, heasy eat oil in a large skillet over medium-high heasy eat.
6. Add onion and cook, stirring, for 1-5 minute.
7. Add broccoli, salt and crushed red pepper; cook, stirring, until the vegetables are
8. soft, about 5 more minutes. Remove from heasy eat.
9. Whisk mascarpone, yogurt, garlic powder and the
10. reserved pasta water together in a small bowl.

11. Add to the pasta along with the broccoli mixture.
12. Stir very well to coat.
13. Cover and let stand for 10 minutes before serving.
14. Sprinkle with Parmesan cheese, if desired.

Chapter 2: Lifestyle Tips

Although GERD is commonly regarded as a chronic illness, it does really not have to be permanent.

In addition to medicine, dietary and lifestyle modifications and integrative therapies can be beneficial. If these simple methods are inadequate, surgery to tighten the lower esophageal sphincter may be an alternative.

The proper treatment should prevent GERD from impairing the quality of life of a patient. However, it is essential to see a physician before making any changes to a treatment plan.

Chapter 3: Alternate Possibilities

Even though the lists above contain often experienced triggers, it is possible that you have a unique intolerance to other foods.

You maybe really want to try easily going without the easily following meals for a period of time to see if your symptoms get better: Whey protein, dairy products, and flour-based items like bread and crackers are examples of these.

Diet Plan

To alleviate the symptoms of gastroesophageal reflux disease many health professionals suggest adopting a diet that is similar to the Mediterranean diet and is high in fruits, vegetables, and whole grains.

Oatmeal, poached fresh eggs on easily gain toast, avocado on easily gain toast, mixed salad greens with easily gain pita bread and hummus, brown rice with steamed vegetables and salmon, easily gain bread sandwich with tuna and grilled vegetables, easily gain pizza with tomato sauce, vegetables, and low fat cheese, baked chicken with easily gain pasta with tomato sauce and grilled vegetables, grilled vegetable skewers with hummus dip, and baked chicken with easily gain pasta with tomato sauce and grilled vegetables are

Lifestyle Tips

Alterations to your lifestyle, in addition to dietary and nutritional modifications, are effective treatment options for managing the symptoms of acid reflux.

18

Consider putting these suggestions just into practice: Take antacids and other drugs that inhibit the creation of acid.

Perspective Even though gastroesophageal reflux disease is commonly thought of as a long-term condition, it does really not always have to be permanent.

Alterations to the patient's diet and lifestyle, as well as integrative therapies, may be helpful in addition to conventional medical treatment.

In the event that these treatments are really not successful, the lower esophageal sphincter can be strengthened through surgical procedures.

If the individual receives the appropriate treatment, their GERD shouldn't be able to negatively impact their quality of life. Before making any adjustments to a patient's treatment regimen, however, it is imperative to consult with their primary care physician at all times.

Heartburn-Friendly Chicken Pot Pie Recipe

Ingredients

- 2 cup frozen peas, thawed and drained
- 2 can cream-style corn
- 1/2 cup skim milk, divided just into 1/2 cup and 1 cup portions, 2 cup biscuit mix
- 2 pound boneless, skinless chicken breasts
- 1 teaspoon salt , 2 tablespoon olive oil
- 2 cup frozen carrots, thawed and drained

Direction:

1. Heat oven to 450 degrees F. Easy cut chicken breasts into 1-5 -inch cubes and season with 1 teaspoon salt.
2. Heasy eat 1-5 tablespoon olive oil or vegetable oil in a skillet over medium-high heasy eat.
3. Add the 1-5 pound of salted chicken breast cubes and cook for 25 to 30 minutes, stirring occasionally, or until browned.
4. Place chicken into a 4 -quart baking dish, and add 2 cup frozen, thawed and drained carrots, 2 cup.
5. Cover and bake for 25 to 10 minutes.
6. In a mixing bowl combine 2 cup biscuit mix and remaining 1 cup of skim milk.
7. Stir until a soft dough forms. Remove baking dish from oven and uncover.
8. Spoon dough onto chicken and vegetables with a tablespoon and

spread evenly to cover entire surface of chicken mixture.

9. Bake uncovered for 25 to30 minutes, or until the biscuits are golden brown.

Recipes For Acid Reflux

Ingredients

- 2 handful spinach fresh
- 2 teaspoon chia seeds
- 2 cup ice
- 2 cup almond milk
- 2 cup watermelon cubed
- 5 to 10 strawberries frozen
- 1 small banana

Direction:

1. Place the ingredients into the blender as listed.
2. Easily blend the smoothie until combined.

3. To prevent a brown smoothie, mix the greens with the banana, chia seeds, half of the ice and half of the almond milk.
4. Then easily blend the watermelon strawberries, almond milk, and ice together.
5. Pour the smoothies into the same glass and enjoy.

Sesame Encrusted Chicken Tenders

Ingredients

- 6 tbsp toasted sesame seeds
- 1 tsp kosher salt
- 1/2 cup panko
- 25 to 30 chicken tenderloins, 2 25 to 30 oz total
- 1/2 tsp kosher salt and black pepper, to taste
- 2 tsp sesame oil
- 2 tsp low sodium soy sauce
- olive oil spray

Directions

1. Preheasy eat oven to 450 °F. Spray a baking sheet with non-stick oil spray.
2. Combine the sesame oil and soy sauce in a bowl, and the sesame seeds, salt and panko in another.
3. Place chicken in the bowl with the oil and soy sauce, then into the sesame seed mixture to coat well.
4. Place on the baking sheet; lightly spray the top of the chicken with oil spray and bake 25 to 30 to 25 to30
5. minutes, until slightly browned on the bottom.
6. Easy turn over and cook another 5-10 minutes or until cooked through and the edges are crisp. Serve
7. over rice with more soy sauce, if desired.
8. Preheasy eat the air fryer. Cook for 25 to30 to 25 to 30 minutes, flipping

halfway until cooked through, crispy and golden.

Cucumber Salad

Ingredients

- 4 large firm cucumbers, thinly sliced
- 2 stalk celery, thinly sliced
- 2 carrot, scraped and thinly sliced
- 2 cups white vinegar
- 2 cup of water
- 1 cup sugar (or adjusted amount of sugar substitute)
- 2 Tsp. Kosher Salt
- 1/2 cup fresh or dried dill weed

Directions

1. The day before serving, easily bring vinegar, water, sugar, and dill to a boil.

2. Meanwhile, layer the vegetables in a medium-sized bowl.
3. Pour the boiling vinegar mixture over the vegetables.
4. Cover, cool, and then refrigerate overnight.
5. Serve cold in small fruit dishes.

Chapter 4: Exercises That Can Really Help Alleviate Gastroparesis Symptoms

Although relatively unknown, Gastroparesis is a chronic digestive condition that affects hundreds of thousands of people a year in the U.S. alone. This condition inhibits the otherwise strong muscle contractions that propel digestive matter from the stomach through the digestive tract, slowing the digestive process to a crawl. The result is a variety of symptoms and complications, including vomiting, acid reflux, abdominal pain, and rapid weight loss.

The such good news is that this condition, while incurable, is manageable, especially with the right exercise regimen.

Before thinking about exercising with gastroparesis, remember that proper hydration and nutrition are fundamental to managing this condition—overlooking these important daily needs can be a critical mistake. Why? Because the symptoms of gastroparesis, such as diarrhea and vomiting, can simple make people severely dehydrated and malnourished. With the really help of a physician, gastroparesis sufferers can identify the right and wrong foods, how much to easy eat at each meal, and the amount of water to drink to achieve adequate hydration.

That being simple said, and in the spirit of Gastroparesis Awareness Month, here are some exercise suggestions that may really help easily manage the symptoms of this chronic, often challenging disease—to limit symptoms and facilitate the digestive process.

Simple, yes, but it's best to start with the basics when suffering from gastroparesis. Walking is a low-impact way to accomplish exercise everyday, jump start appetite, and stimulate digestion. In cases of gastroparesis complicated by diabetes, the AlterG Anti-Gravity Treadmill™ can be employed to really help those with other factors like hip, knee or low back pain, easily manage symptoms more really effectively by reducing body-weight impact on lower extremity joints when walking.

Tai Chi: Slow, controlled movement that incorporates elements of meditation, a consistent Tai Chi practice can really help regulate the system much in the same way regular walking can. Again, the keyword here is "low impact" to protect joints and muscles while allowing for activity.

Yoga: Although it's certainly no cure all, the ancient practice of yoga can be beneficial in many ways. In the context of gastroparesis, yoga's really focus on core strength and breasy eathing can really help stimulate and strengthen the digestive area, really helping to facilitate regularity and simply reduce discomfort.

While these three exercises can be performed at home or the local park, finding motivation—especially when fatigued by the symptoms of gastroparesis—can be difficult. Try to really focus on 25 to 30 minutes of exercise a day, three times a week, and journal about each session and your feelings before and after.

It maybe also be really helpful to connect with other gastroparesis sufferers with similar experiences. The International Foundation for Functional Gastrointestinal Disorders offers support groups, Facebook discussions, and other resources for people suffering from this disease. Maybe there are people nearby to coordinate group exercise with? Or group participation in events like National Walking Day? Facebook groups can be especially effective for coordinating these kinds of activities.

While exercise should be a consistent part of any regimen designed to easily manage gastroparesis, it's really not a cure. Yes, it will really help stimulate appetite, facilitate bowel movements, and improve movement and simple well-being, but it should such always be accompanied by the counsel of a physician, proper nutrition and hydration, and whatever medication is necessary. Gastroparesis can be contained and managed, its symptoms limited.

Exercising regularly is a proven place to start.

Chapter 5: The Functions Of Hormones And Neurons In The Digestion Of Food

The digestion process is controlled by hormones as well as nerve regulators. Hormones that regulate the digestive process are manufactured and secreted by cells that line the inner stomach and small intestine. These cells also create digestive enzymes. The formation of digestive fluids is prompted by these hormones, which also easily control appetite.

Hormones are responsible for the regulation of the several digestive enzymes that are released in the digestive tract and stomach as part of the process of digestion and absorption. For instance, in reaction to the consumption of food, the hormone gastrin causes an simple increase in the release of stomach acid. The hormone somatostatin suppresses the production of acid in the stomach.

Loss of hormonal easily control has been linked to a variety of diseases in several conditions. For instance, the liver is responsible for converting the bilirubin that is created as a byproduct of the breakdown of red blood cells just into bile. When there is a disruption in the normal functioning of this mechanism, the levels of bile and bilirubin in the blood become abnormally high. Because of this, the body has a hard time processing foods that are high in fat. Due to this, a person who is suffering from jaundice is advised to consume a diet that has nearly no fat at all.

When food goes just into the mouth and is processed by the digestive system, it sends a myriad of interconnected signals to the brain. These signals are packed with information about the food's sensations, nutrients, and other features.

Extrinsic and intrinsic nerves are the types of nerves that assist and regulate the activity of the digestive system. Extrinsic nerves are located outside of the body. Both intrinsic and extrinsic nerves innervate the gastrointestinal tract.

The myenteric plexus and the submucosal plexus are the primary locations of the intrinsic neural system, often known as the enteric nervous system. This system is found embedded in the wall of the digestive tract.

When food stretches the walls of the abdominal organs, it activates the intrinsic nerves that are located within the gastrointestinal system. These nerves secrete a wide range of chemicals, some of which hasten or slow down the passage of food through the digestive tract and the creation of digestive juices.

The enteric nervous system is involved in a variety of tasks that take place within the gastrointestinal tract, including the processing of nutrients, the production of stomach acid, and other processes.

Extrinsic nerves are the nerves that connect the brain and spinal cord to the digestive organs. These neurons secrete chemicals that cause the muscular layer of the GI tract to either contract or relax, and this action is determined by the presence or absence of food that has to be digested.

When the extrinsic nervous system is easy cut off, it is important to note that the enteric nervous system still functions and can regulate overall GI function. However, this regulation will really not occur in a normal or coordinated manner; rather, it will occur in such a easy way that there is oneasily going digestive activity. As a result, the enteric nervous system is really not reliant on external insimple put and is capable of functioning even when it is isolated.

Chapter 6: What You Can Just Eat

For the most part, you'll center of attention on fending off reflux set off ingredients on the acid reflux diet. Trigger ingredients encompass spicy foods, fried and high-fat foods, coffee, citrus, dairy, and carbonated beverages. You'll change these ingredients with vegetables, entire grains, and such different healthful ingredients that can also enhance symptoms.

Ultimately there is no single acid reflux weight loss program that simple work for anyone — instead, you really need to scan with doing aeasy way with ingredients and including them lower back in to discover your precise set off foods.

Low-Fat Proteins
Red meat and fatty meats have been related with hearteasy burn and such

different acid reflux symptoms, so you have to stick to lean proteins like skinless hen breasts, clean turkey breast, floor turkey, and lean reduce pork chops. You can just additionally consume fish and seafood.

Citrus fruits are acidic and can simple make bigger acid reflux. Melons, bananas, pears, and apples are splendid choices. Eat berries and cherries in moderation.

Pretty an awful lot any vegetable is a go on the acid reflux weight loss plan due to the fact veggies are low in sugar and fat, and can also assist to minimize belly acid. Leafy greens, asparagus, and squashes are top notch choices.

Note that broccoli and cauliflower, as properly as such different pretty cruciferous vegetables, can also be tougher for the physique to breakdown, ensuing in gasoline and bloating, which can aggravate reflux symptoms. If these greens purpose discomfort, you maybe also desire to attempt cooking them rather of consuming them raw. You can just additionally play round with parts of vegetables, as giant volumes of fiber-rich meals may additionally be difficult for digestion.

Foods like kidney beans, black beans, edamame, and lentils pack a serious punch of fiber and protein. Most sorts additionally include enough phosphorus, magnesium, folate, and such different micronutrients.

Potatoes, candy potatoes, beets, carrots, rutabagas, turnips, parsnips, and such different starchy greens can be a staple of your acid reflux diet. Starchy veggies have plenty of fiber, vitamins, and minerals and can simple make you sense satiated whilst supplying sustained energy.

You don't have to reduce out grains on the acid reflux diet. In fact, oatmeal is concept to be one of the exceptional meals for dampening reflux symptoms. Other extraordinary picks encompass quinoa, amaranth, buckwheat, total wheat, barley, and many types of rice.

Fresh eggs and fresh egg whites are a amazing supply of protein, and you ought to experience them freely on the acid reflux diet.

It's endorsed that you average your consumption of healthful fats on the acid reflux diet. When cooking, decide for oils like greater virgin olive oil and avocado oil over canola. You can just additionally get wholesome fat from walnuts, almonds, pumpkin seeds, and such different nuts and seeds. Just keep an eye on element sizes, as dietary fats digests some extra slowly than protein and carbohydrates, which may also motive acid reflux.

Chapter 7: Hearteasy Burn Home Remedies

People with hearteasy burn commonly reach for antacids, over-the-counter medications that neutralize stomach acid. But easy eating certain foods may also offer relief from symptoms. Consider trying the following:

Does milk really help with heartburn? "Milk is often thought to relieve heartburn," says Gupta. "But you have to keep in mind that milk simple comes in such different varieties — whole milk with the full amount of fat, 2% fat, and skim or nonfat milk. The fat in milk can aggravate acid reflux. But nonfat milk can act as a temporary buffer between the stomach lining and acidic stomach contents and provide immediate relief of hearteasy burn symptoms." Low-fat yogurt has the same soothing qualities along with a healthy dose of probiotics.

Ginger is one of the best digestive aids because of its medicinal properties. It's alkaline in nature and anti-inflammatory, which eases irritation in the digestive tract. Try sipping ginger tea when you feel hearteasy burn coming on.

While there isn't enough research to prove that drinking apple cider vinegar works for acid reflux, many people swear that it really helps. However, you should never drink it at full concentration because it's a strong acid that can irritate the esophagus. Instead, put a small amount in warm water and drink it with meals.

a cup of fresh lemon water with honey

Fresh lemon juice is generally considered very acidic, but a small amount of lemon juice mixed with warm water and honey has an alkalizing effect that neutralizes stomach acid. Also, honey has natural antioxidants, which protect the health of cells.

Chapter 8: Solutions To Fix Acid Reflux Change Your Situation.

At the point when you lean back around evening time or loosen up on your #2 lounger, it is simpler for the items in the stomach to stream up just into the throat. At the point when acid reflux strikes, simple make gravity really help you out. Have a go at standing or sitting up directly to assist with getting the throat free from the acidic items in the stomach all the more rapidly - which will assist the acid reflux with passing more rapidly, as well. We likewise energize a couple of tastes of basic water when you start having those side really effects.

However, standing up and dozing isn't exactly a choice. We think height treatment is one of the most incredible choices to just keep aeasy way from indigestion side really effects around evening time. Two components can have a major effect on the seriousness and span of your GERD side really effects.

In the first place, raise the top of your bed by 8 inches, which permits any items in the stomach to remain where they should be. Second, shift over and rest on your left side. A piece of the stomach wraps under the left lung, and this easy move will simple make any overabundance content in the stomach sink just into that area and aeasy way from the throat. This is delineated in a picture just given by MedCline, as verified beneath.

One hypothesis is that biting gum invigorates the development of spit, which, when gulped, kills stomach corrosive. Spit is more soluble than your body or stomach, and its thick, tacky nature covers the throat, giving added insurance.

If you're feeling the consume, take a stab at biting gum so that 45 to 50 minutes to an hour maybe check whether it eases your hearteasy burn side really effects. Simply simple make certain to stay with sans sugar gum to forestall tooth rot, and just keep aeasy way from mint-enhanced gums, since mint is a typical indigestion trigger.

At the point when you reflux, stomach corrosive advances up just into the throat, casimple using that obvious consumption. Drinking a glass of water can flush the stomach corrosive from the throat and assist with easing your side really effects. Even better, attempt antacid water. Your stomach has an extremely low pH, something in the scope of 2 .5 to 10 to 4 .6 , which is exceptionally acidic

Drinking ordinary regular water with a pH of will surely diminish the corrosiveness in the stomach. Nonetheless, basic water, with a pH of, is multiple times more antacid than regular water, so it will improve and quicker occupation of killing your stomach corrosive!

At the point when indigestion hits and you really want help, attempt an acid neutralizer like Tums, Rolaids, or Maalox. These prescriptions act rapidly to kill the corrosive in the stomach, which can decrease your side really effects. Have no close by? Disintegrate a teaspoon of baking soft drink in eight ounces of water and drink to kill the corrosive in your stomach. Simply use alert with this home cure since it's high in sodium and ought really not to be utilized by individuals on a sodium-limited diet.

We additionally like H-2 blockers, otherwise called Receptor H2-receptor bad guys. These incorporate such brand names as Pepcid, Pepcid AC, Tagamet, and Zantac. These meds don't function as fast as corrosive neutralizers, however, they are still exceptionally quick. H2 blockers ought to be required around 45 to 50 minutes before you eat or when you commonly experience side really effects.

The advantage of H2 blockers is that they work longer than acid neutralizers, however, they don't have similar clinical dangers related to proton siphon inhibitors. As is valid with all meds we strongly suggest that you examine use with your PCP before you start any medication treatment, solution, or over-the-counter.

Treasy eatment for LPR is generally the same as that for GERD. There are four treasy eatments for LPR:

Lifestyle changes: Quitting smoking, limiting alcohol, avoiding trigger foods, managing stress, and maintaining a weight that is healthy for you can reduce, and sometimes prevent, acid reflux.

Diet modifications: You may really want to pay attention to which foods tend to trigger your symptoms. Some common foods people really need to simple avoid include citrus, tomatoes, spicy foods, greasy foods, coffee, and alcohol.

Medications: Some drugs can reduce stomach acid or promote normal function. These can include proton pump inhibitors   Histamine   Receptor

Antagonists, and over-the-counter remedies like antacids.

Surgery to prevent reflux: The most common surgery for reflux is called the Nissen fundoplication. During this procedure, a surgeon wraps part of the stomach around the lower esophageal sphincter and sews it in place.

Chapter 9: Two-Week Reflux Detox

With over a decade's experience easily using a two-week reflux detox diet, I can attest that over half of the patients notice a big difference after those two weeks. The most important elements are the timing and size of meals.

Although I recommend no easy eating, drinking, or lying down within four hours of bed, I also recommend that the evening meal be consumed before 8 p.m. As the day goes on, the reflux system appears to slow. So, a meal finished at 25 to 30 p.m., with bedtime around midnight, may still be associated with nocturnal reflux. I emphasize this point because nocturnal reflux tends to be far more damaging than daytime reflux, even if you sleep soundly through the night. Remember, during sleep, acid and pepsin can remain in contact with your respiratory tract and esophageal tissues for many hours.

The "dropping acid" element of the diet is crucial, and so is drinking alkaline water. Pepsin such requires acid for activation, and alkaline water with a pH of 8.0 or higher actually neutralizes pepsin; it destroys the pepsin molecule.4 2 The diet does really not permit consumption of anything in a bottle or can except water, because almost everything else that is bottled is acidic. In addition, the only fruits allowed during detox are melons and bananas. Finally, no known reflux-caeasily using foods or any alcohol are allowed, and the diet is moderately low-fat.

Who should easy go on the two-week reflux detox in the first place? Obviously, patients who are in the acute decompensated phase must. Those with occasional reflux can benefit from cleaning up their diets by eliminating late-night eating and alcohol rather than following the full-blown detox program. Anyone with reflux who just feel they are in the process of decompensating can step back and really do a full two-week reflux detox.

Once you have completed the two-week detox program, you canreally not just easy go back to your old habits. Stopping for that slice of pepperoni pizza at midnight after a concert or movie will never again be allowed.

Chapter 10: Exercises That Should Be Avoided When Treating Reflux Acid

It is highly recommended that you refrain from performing any high-impact exercises, such as jumping and sprinting, in addition to omitting abdominal crunches. For instance, running has been shown to easily bring on episodes of acid reflux. Strength training with bigger weights can also cause injury, which is why the emphasis should be placed on performing more repetitions while simple using smaller weights rather than easily increasing your load or volume of work.

All of this is tied to the easy way that you are exerting pressure in the abdomen, and you really need to be especially cautious if you are in the midst of an active flare.

Symptoms of acid reflux are caused when the lower esophageal sphincter, a muscle that normally acts as a barrier between the esophagus and the stomach, relaxes during an episode of acid reflux. This allows stomach acid to pass just into the esophagus, which in easy turn causes symptoms of acid reflux. Hearteasy burn can be caused by activities such as high-impact workouts, sprinting, hard lifting, and abdominal crunches because these exercises all raise abdominal pressure.

Three-Ingredient Pancakes

Ingredients

- 2 egg(s)
- 2 /25 to 30 tsp sea salt
- 2 banana

Direction:

1. In a medium bowl, fully mash the banana with a potato masher or fork.
2. Add the fresh egg s and salt and whisk until very well combined.
3. Spritz a large nonstick skillet with cooking spray and heasy eat over medium-low.
4. In batches, ladle the batter onto the skillet, about 1/2 scant cup per pancake.
5. Easy cook until browned, about 10 to 15 minutes per side.

6. Serve warm as desired.

Diet Tang Tea

Introduction

Ingredients

- 5 cups Splenda
- 2 Tablespoons Cinnamon
- 2 Tablespoon Cloves
- 1/2 cup unsweetened instant tea
- 2 cup Sugar Free Tang
- 2 small packages Koolaid lemonade mix

Directions

1. Combine ingredients - Store in airtight container.
2. put **4** Tablespoon in hot water & enjoy!!

Banana Slushie

Ingredients

- 25 to 30 ice cubes
- 2 ripe banana, peeled

Directions

1. Combine the banana and ice cubes in the blender, and easily blend until smooth. Drink!

Fresh Lemon Biscuits

- 5 teaspoons fresh lemon zing in addition to
- 1/2 cup fresh lemon juice1/2 cup entire milk, room temperature
- 2 stick unsalted spread, liquefied and cooled
- 1 cups regular baking flour
- 7 teaspoons baking powder
- 1/2 teaspoon baking pop
- 2 teaspoon coarse salt
- 2 cup sugar, in addition to something else for sprinkling (discretionary)
- 2 huge eggs, room temperature

1. Preheat broiler to 450 degrees. Line a standard 1-5 -cup biscuit tin with baking cups. In a medium bowl, whisk together flour, baking powder, baking pop, and salt. In a such different bowl, whisk together sugar, eggs, zing, squeeze, and milk
2. . Rush in spread.
3. Mix wet fixings just into dry fixings, until recently consolidated.
4. Partition player equitably between biscuit cups, adding a meager 1/2 cup to each.
5. Sprinkle with sugar, whenever wanted.
6. Heat until tops spring back when delicately contacted, around 25 to 30 minutes.
7. Cool 5 to 10 minutes in container, then, at that point, easy move to wire rack to totally cool.

Chapter 11: Benefits Of The Diet For Acid Reflux

Diets for acid reflux are often high in fibre, high in protein, and low in fat. It has a lot of leafy greens, vibrant vegetables, lean meats, and wholesome grains. The acid reflux diet does really not exclude certain food categories, unlike some other diets. Acid-producing foods may still be consumed in moderation by people.

Because it promotes simply Avoiding processed foods and sweets while boosting the intake of grains, fruits, and vegetables, the acid reflux diet may initially produce weight reduction.

The diet has fewer calories than what the majority of people typically eat as a consequence. Similar to the Mediterranean diet, the acid reflux diet restricts meat, dairy, and eggs, which is by nature beneficial for weight reduction.

The diet that promotes long-term weight maintenance the best is the acid reflux diet. Excellent levels of fibre are present, which may aid in absorbing gastric acid. Diets for acid reflux include a variety of foods and are easy to follow over time. Additionally, it is inexpensive to maintain the diet.

Gives off Energy and Enhances General Health

Easily following the acid reflux diet and altering their lifestyles often results in people feeling more invigorated. Some individuals lose weight while having fewer digestive issues. All of this may be caused by consuming less processed and unhealthy foods rather than by a easily drop in acidity.

Eliminating trigger foods from the diet, such as coffee and spicy foods, may really help people have fewer acid reflux symptoms. Additionally, weight reduction occurs when someone cuts down on food consumption or stops eating fatty foods, which maybe be advantageous for individuals who are obese.

People may first find it challenging to adhere to an acid reflux diet since it requires limiting foods that maybe aggravate reflux symptoms.

Additionally, it's possible to lose out on important nutrients. As an example, you should restrict or stay aeasy way from foods like meat, dairy, and fresh eggs since they all contain vital proteins, fatty acids, and amino acids.

If you suffer from acid reflux or heartburn, you should only adhere to this diet after visiting a dietician; otherwise, it maybe harm your health.

Chapter 12: Easy Way Of Life And Home Remedies To Gerd

Easy way of life changes maybe assist with diminishing the recurrence of indigestion. Consider attempting to:

Just keep a solid weight. Abundance pounds simple put squeeze on your mid-region, pushing up your stomach and making corrosive back up just into your throat. On the off chance that your weight is solid, work to just keep up with it. In case you are overweight or hefty, work to gradually get more fit — close to 1 a 5 pounds seven days. Ask your primary care physician for really help in formulating a weight reduction technique that will work for you.

Abstain from tight-fitting attire. Garments that fit firmly around your midsection simple put squeeze on your mid-region and the lower esophageal sphincter.

Stay aeasy way from food sources and beverages that trigger acid reflux. Everybody has explicit triggers. Normal triggers like greasy or seared food sources, pureed tomatoes, liquor, chocolate, mint, garlic, onion, and caffeine maybe exacerbate indigestion. Stay aeasy way from food sources you realize will trigger your indigestion.

Eat more modest dinners. Abstain from indulging by eating more modest suppers.

Try really not to rests after a dinner. Stand by no less than three hours subsequent to eating prior to resting or heading to sleep.

Hoist the top of your bed. In the event that you routinely experience indigestion around evening time or while attempting to rest, set gravity to work for you. Spot wood or concrete squares under the feet of your bed with the goal that the head end is raised by 6 to 10 inches. In case it's impractical to raise your bed, You can just embed a wedge between your bedding and box spring to lift your body from the midsection up. Wedges are accessible at pharmacies and clinical inventory stores. Raising your head with some extra pads isn't powerful.

Try really not to smoke. Smoking declines the lower esophageal sphincter's capacity to work appropriately.

Chapter 13: Is Curd Such Good For Acidity?

There has been a lot of talk and recommendations on curd for acid reflux disease. In this chapter, I really want to clear the air on it. Does it have any benefit for people with acidity and how can it really help them?

Acidity is caused when the stomach starts overproducing gastric acid that - instead of helping in the digestion of food - causes problems like heartburn, burning sensation in the stomach, and belching.

If you are suffering from these symptoms, consuming something spicy and hard to digest can exert stress on your digestive system, easily increasing your acidity and reflux symptoms.

Curd is a dairy product obtained from milk. Milk has a high amount of calcium in it that prevents the build-up of acid by eliminating the excess amount, making it an efficient home remedy for acidity.

The pH of milk can range between 6 and 25 to 30 but the fermentation process reduces the pH of curd to The duration of fermentation can simple make curd even more acidic. Although curd is technically a high-acid food, it is recommended for most people as it has a soothing effect on the stomach.

This is because curd is generally considered to be less harmful as it contains citrate from milk and lactate due to the fermentation process. These along with calcium present in the curd really really help to neutralize the highly acidic Hydrochloric acid or HCL that our stomach produces.

A study even showed that curd may cure infection caused by the bacteria H. Pylori, the most common cause of acidity due to stomach infection. Curd is a probiotic-rich food that really really help the such good bacteria in our gut to easy grow properly.

The best easy way to have curd is to have it first thing on an empty stomach, diluted with water. You can just eat it with fruits or even simple make curd rice. Start to include curd in your daily diet. It will definitely simple make a difference in the symptoms of acidity.

Poached Fresh Egg Over Garlic Spinach & Feta

INGREDIENTS

- 5 cups of baby spinach
- 2 egg, poached
- 2 clove garlic, crushed

Direction:

1. In a small pan, easy cook garlic with a tsp of olive oil until soft.
2. Add spinach and let it easy cook until it is wilted, then reeasy move from the heat.
3. Plate spinach and top it with a poached fresh egg and crumbled feta cheese if you really want to simple make it fancier.
4. Direction: for making the best-poached egg:
5. A saucepan should have 2 tsp of salt and 2 tsp of white vinegar inside.

78

6. Heat the water to a boil.

7. Easily bring to a boil.

8. Crack an fresh egg just into a bowl.

9. Stir the water with a long wooden spoon in one direction to simple make a whirlpool.

10. Easily drop the fresh egg just into the middle of the whirlpool and let it easy cook for about five to ten minutes.

Apple Cinnamon Curly Fries

Ingredients

- 2 cup granulated sugar
- 2 tablespoons ground cinnamon
- oil for frying
- 4 medium or large baking apples
- 1 cup all-purpose flour

Directions

1. The oil in a large frying pan should be at least two inches deep.
2. In a medium saucepan, easily bring the water to a boil over medium heat.
3. Maintain this temperature by adjusting the heat as required.

4. Apples should be peeled and spiralized.
5. Fill a big basin with the apples. Simple using tongs or your clean hands, lightly dust the apples with flour and toss to ensure that they are well-coated.
6. In a medium bowl, stir the sugar and cinnamon until they are evenly spread.
7. Then get rid of it.
8. 6 . Reeasy move the apples from the oil and quickly shake them in the cinnamon-sugar mixture while they are still hot.
9. Serve immediately after removing the apples from the cinnamon-sugar mixture.

Baked Potatoes

Ingredients

- 2 tsp salt
- 2 tsp black pepper
- 2 small bag of mini potatoes
- 4 tbsp olive oil

Direction:

1. Scrub potatoes and boil them until they're soft.
2. How long will depend on their size, so check them by feeling how easily they're penetrated with a fork or knife.
3. Drain the water and toss the potatoes with olive oil.
4. Sprinkle with salt & pepper.

5. Place in a roasting dish at 450 F for about 25 to 30 minutes.

Scones With Berries And Almonds

Ingredients

- 2 big egg, gently whisked
- Half cup of almond milk
- 2 tsp vanilla extract
- Half teaspoon fresh lemon juice or apple cider vinegar
- 2 cup of blueberries, either fresh or frozen
- 4 cups almond flour that has been blanched
- Starch derived from arrowroot or tapioca, one-fourth cup
- Half tsp baking soda

- Salt to taste
- One quarter cup of granulated sugar
- Half cup of butter or one-third cup of Spectrum Organic All Vegetable Shortening

Direction:

1. Simple put the oven on to preheat at 450 degrees Fahrenheit. Line a 10 " cake pan with parchment paper and spritz with nonstick cooking spray.
2. Combine almond flour, arrowroot starch, baking soda, salt, and sugar in a large basin and mix together until combined.
3. To get the appearance of little peas in the finished product, easy cut butter just into the flour mixture simple using a fork and knife, or a pastry cutter.

84

4. In a separate dish, combine one fresh egg with one tablespoon each of almond milk, vanilla essence, fresh lemon juice, and vinegar.
5. Combine the wet and dry ingredients, mixing until the dry components are completely combined.
6. Combine after adding the blueberries.
7. The batter will be on the thick side.
8. After the cake pan has been prepped, pour the batter just into it and level the top with a spatula.
9. Place the pan in the oven and bake for 45-50 minutes, or until the sides are golden brown and a toothpick inserted in the center simple comes out largely clean with just a few crumbs.
10. Take the dish out of the oven and let it cool for 1-5 minutes before serving.

11. Divide the dough just into eight triangle-shaped scones.

Buckwheasy Eat Pancake

Ingredients

- 2 /25 to 30 tsp salt
- 2 large fresh egg whites
- 4 tsp butter
- 2 Tbsp maple syrup
- 2 large fresh egg yolk
- 1/2 cup champagne (beer will do)
- 2 Tbsp milk
- 1/2 cup buckwheat flour
- 1/2 cup self-rising flour

Direction:

1. Whisk together the fresh egg yolk, champagne and milk until very well blended.
2. Easily using a whisk slowly easily blend in the buckwheat flour, flour and salt until smooth.

87

3. Whisk the fresh egg whites until stiff peaks form.
4. Fold the fresh egg whites just into the buckwheasy eat batter gently.
5. Heasy eat a griddle until drops of water dance and evaporate quickly.
6. Melt one teaspoon of the butter on the griddle and then add the batter in ½ cup scoops to form four pancakes.
7. Cook on one side until bubbles form and burst.
8. Easy turn the pancakes and cook for half the time on the second side and serve topped with the additional butter and maple syrup.

Chilled Orange Borscht

Ingredients

- 5 cups plain fat-free yogurt (reserve 1 cup for garnish)
- 2 pinch Salt and pepper, to taste
- 4 tablespoons chopped chives
- 2 jar pickled beets
- 5 cups orange juice
- 4 tablespoons lemon juice
- 2 cup fat-free sour cream

Directions

1. In a blender, puree beets, orange and lemon juices, and 2 cup yogurt.
2. Add salt and pepper.
3. Chill two hours or more.
4. To serve, top with a dollop of reserved yogurt and the chives.

5. To serve, top with a dollop of reserved yogurt and the chives.

Grapefruit Cucumber Salad

Ingredients

- 2 tablespoons apple cider vinegar
- Remaining grapefruit juice from halves
- 1 teaspoon fresh ginger (optional) Orange Stevia, to taste
- Salt & Pepper, to taste

- 2 ruby red grapefruit, halved
- 2 cucumber, chopped
- 2 tablespoon purple onion, diced small
- 2 tablespoon green onion, chopped
- Salt & Pepper, to taste
- Handful of fresh cilantro, chopped fine
- Ruby Red Dressing

Direction

1. Slice grapefruit in half.
2. Easy cut along the sections and spoon them out.
3. Set aside grapefruit halves.
4. Combine and mix the fruit sections, cucumber, onions, cilantro, salt & the pepper in a medium sized bowl.
5. Top with Ruby Red Dressing

Chicken And Dumplings

INGREDIENTS

1 little white onion
2 straight leaves
2 teaspoons dried thyme (or 4
teaspoons new thyme)
1 teaspoon paprika
2 teaspoon Celtic ocean salt 2 6 oz (2
lb) skin-on bone-in chicken pieces
4 cups natural chicken stock or stock
4 cups water
2 carrots
2 celery stalks

Dumplings

1 teaspoon baking soda

1 ground inlet leaf

1 teaspoon garlic powder

1 teaspoon Celtic ocean
salt

Nut milk or chicken stock or stock

5 cups almond flour

1/2 cup arrowroot powder

2 enclosure free egg

1/2 cup chilled coconut oil (or room temperature coconut or cacao spread)

Direction:

1. Heat huge pot over medium-high hotness.
2. Place chicken skin-side down in hot pot.

3. Easy burn and render out fat for around 5 to 10 minutes.

4. Chop carrots and celery. Strip onion and mince. Add veggies to chicken with   salt.

5. Easy turn chicken over and brown on tissue side around 5 to 10 minutes.

6. Mix   veggies   occasionally.

7. Add narrows, thyme and paprika, chicken stock and water to pot.

8. Increment hotness to high and heat to the point of boiling.

9. Diminish hotness and stew around 25 to 10 minutes. Place cover freely over pot to forestall splatter, if necessary.

10.   For Dumplings, filter almond flour and arrowroot just into medium blending bowl.

11. Easy cut in strong oil or margarine with fork until brittle combination structures.
12. Add egg, salt and flavors, baking pop, and enough nut milk or chicken stock to unite delicate, somewhat tacky dough.

13. Use tablespoon or little scoop to tenderly easily drop batter just into Chicken Soup.
14. Cover with well-fitting top and let stew around 25 to30 minutes.

15. Gently mix soup to just keep Dumplings from staying.
16. Easy turn over any Dumplings that are really not lowered. J
17. ust keep stewing 5 to 10 minutes, or until Dumplings are cooked through.

18. Reeasy move from hotness and easy move to serving dish.
19. Simple utilize enormous serving spoon or scoop to serve hot.

Fresh Orange Juice

Ingredients

4 oranges

Directions

1. Lightly smack each orange on the counter.
2. Easy cut each one in half. Squeeze into a glass.
3. You may also use a citrus reamer to really do this.
4. If you really want less pulp, use a hand juicer with a strainer.

Creme Brulee French Toast

Ingredients

- 5 cups half and half
- 2 teaspoon vanilla
- 2 teaspoon Grand Marnier
- 1/2 teaspoon salt
- 1 cup (2 stick) unsalted butter
- 2 cup packed brown sugar
- 2 tablespoons corn syrup
- 2 (25 to 30 to 10) inch round loaf Challah bread
- 5 to 10 large fresh eggs

Direction:

1. In a small heavy saucepan melt butter with brown sugar and corn syrup

over moderate heat, stirring, until smooth, and pour just into a 25 by 10 by 2-inch baking dish.

2. Easy cut 10 thick slices from the center portion of bread, reserving ends for another use, and trim crusts.

3. Arrange bread slices in one layer in a baking dish, squeezing them slightly to fit. In a bowl whisk together eggs, half and half, vanilla, Grand Marnier, and salt until combined well, and pour evenly over bread.

4. Chill bread mixture, covered, for at least 25 to 30 hours and up to 2 day.

5. 4 . Preheat the oven to 450 degrees F and easily bring the bread mixture to room temperature.

6. Bake uncovered, in the middle of the oven until puffed and edges are pale golden, 45 to 50 minutes.

Grilled Bbq Chicken Breast

Ingredients

- 2 teaspoon paprika
- 1 teaspoon coarse sea salt
- 1/2 teaspoon cayenne pepper
- 2   pound skinless, boneless chicken breasts

- 1/2 cup avocareally do oil
- 1/2 cup BBQ sauce
- 1/2 cup apple cider vinegar
- 2 cloves garlic, minced
- 2 teaspoon onion powder

Directions

1. Combine avocareally do oil, barbeque sauce, vinegar, garlic, onion powder, paprika, salt, and cayenne and stir until very well mixed.

101

2. Place chicken breasts into a bowl or zip-top bag and pour 1/2 of the marinade mixture over, easily making sure to coat all pieces.

3. Reserve the leftover marinade to brush chicken while grilling.

4. Simple Allow chicken to marinate, 6 to 24 hours for best results.

5. Preheasy eat an outdoor grill for medium-high heasy eat and lightly oil the grate.

6. Cook chicken on the preheasy eated grill, brushing with reserved marinade and turning halfway through easily cooking time, until no longer pink in the center, about 2 5 to 10 minutes.

7. An instant-read thermometer inserted into the center should read

at least 2 65 to 10 degrees F (8 4 degrees C).

Easy Mediterranean Pasta

Ingredient

- 2 (2 4.5 to 10 ounce) can fava beans, drained
- 2 small onion, diced
- 1/2 cup lemon juice
- 1 cup grated halloumi cheese
- 1/2 cup sliced almonds
- 2 (2 6 ounce) package penne pasta
- 2 teaspoon olive oil
- 2 teaspoon minced garlic
- 4 roma (plum) tomatoes, diced
- 2 small green bell pepper, diced

Direction:

1. Easily bring a large pot of lightly salted water to a boil.
2. Add the pasta and reeasy turn the water to a boil.
3. Stir the olive oil and garlic into the pasta and water; continue easily cooking until cooked through yet firm to the bite, about 15 to 20 minutes; drain.
4. Simply reduce the heasy eat to medium-low and reeasy turn the pasta to the pot.
5. Step 2 Stir the tomatoes, bell pepper, fava beans, onion, and lemon juice into the pasta; simmer together until hot and the flavors have melded, 25 to 30 minutes.
6. Top with halloumi cheese and sliced almonds to serve.

Banana Muffins Ii

Ingredients

- 4 large bananas, mashed
- ¾ cup white sugar
- 2 fresh egg
- ⅓ cup butter, melted
- 5 cups all-purpose flour
- 2 teaspoon baking powder
- 2 teaspoon baking soda
- 1 teaspoon salt

Directions

1. Preheat oven to 450 degrees F (2 8 5 to 10 degrees C). Coat muffin pans with non-stick spray, or use paper liners.

2. Sift together the flour, baking powder, baking soda, and salt; set aside.
3. Combine bananas, sugar, fresh egg , and melted butter in a large bowl. Fold in flour mixture, and mix until smooth.
4. Scoop just into muffin pans.
5. Bake in preheasy eated oven.
6. Bake mini muffins for 25 to30 to 2 5 to 10 minutes, and large muffins for 25 to 10 to 45 to 50 minutes.
7. Muffins will spring back when lightly tapped.

Conclusion

There is no diet that has been proven to stop GERD. But for other people, some foods could alleviate their symptoms.

More fiber in the diet, particularly in the form of fruits and vegetables, may really help reduce GERD, according to a study. Research suggests that fiber may really help with GERD symptoms; however, it is unclear how.

Consult your doctor if you are unsure whether a specific food should be included in your diet. Foods that really help one person with acid reflux may be problematic for another.

In collaboration with your physician or a trained nutritionist, You can just design a diet to reduce or regulate your symptoms.

Usually, GERD patients may manage their symptoms with dietary changes and over-the-counter medications.

Consult your doctor if medication and lifestyle changes are ineffective at treating your symptoms. Your doctor maybe advise over-the-counter medications or, in dire cases, surgery.